HIV AIDS

By
Paula Johanson

16
EasyRead Large

RHYW

Copyright Page from the Original Book

To the girl who roller-skated into my local health center, downstairs, on the Tuesday night clinic for STD and birth control counseling; and to Evelyn, the first of my friends to die of AIDS

Published in 2007 by The Rosen Publishing Group, Inc.
29 East 21st Street, New York, NY 10010

First Edition

Library of Congress Cataloging-in-Publication Data

Johanson, Paula.
HIV and AIDS / Paula Johanson.—1st ed.
p. cm.—(Coping in a changing world)
Includes index.
ISBN-13: 978-1-4042-0948-0 (library binding)
ISBN-10: 1-4042-0948-4 (library binding)
1. AIDS (Diseases)—Juvenile literature.
2. HIV (Viruses)—Juvenile literature. I. Title.
RA643.8.J64 2007
362.196'9792—dc22

2006027075

Manufactured in the United States of America

This optimized ReadHowYouWant edition contains the complete, unabridged text of the original publisher's edition. Other aspects of the book may vary from the original edition.

Published in 2008 in the US and world markets by ReadHowYouWant.

The text in this edition has been formatted and typeset to make reading easier and more enjoyable for ALL kinds of readers. In addition the text has been formatted to the specifications indicated on the title page. The formatting of this edition is the copyright of Objective Systems Pty Ltd.

Set in 16 pt. Verdana

TABLE OF CONTENTS

To the girl who roller-skated into my local health center, downstairs, on the Tuesday night clinic for STD and birth control counseling; and to Evelyn, the first of my friends to die of AIDS

CHAPTER ONE

Discovery and Definition

IT IS THE WORST AND DEADLIEST DISEASE THAT HUMANKIND HAS EVER EXPERIENCED.

If you began asking questions about AIDS, you would probably find that you could get some useful answers about the disease from someone you know—a parent, teacher, friend, or sibling. But you need to know more than just a little about AIDS (acquired immunodeficiency syndrome) and the virus that causes it, HIV (human immunodeficiency virus). You need to know what to do to protect yourself.

The Joint United Nations Program on HIV/AIDS estimates that there were 40.3 million people around the world living with HIV at the end of 2005. Of these, approximately 1.2 million lived in the United States. Sadly, each year more people become infected with the virus, and others who were already infected die from AIDS. Since it was first recognized in 1981, AIDS has killed 25 million people*. "It is the worst and deadliest disease that humankind has ever experienced," according to Mark Stirling, UNAIDS director of East and Southern Africa.** What's worse, there is no cure for or vaccine against AIDS.

[* UNAIDS/WHO AIDS Epidemic Update: December 2005 (http://www.unaids.org/epi/2005/doc/EPIupdate2005_html_en/epi05_03_en.htm).]

[** Associated Press, "AIDS Relentless March Leaves Legacy of Misery," June 5, 2006 (http://www.msnbc.msn.com/id/13072820).]

Although these statistics are frightening, fighting the disease can begin with you. It is true that HIV/AIDS is a growing danger for everyone, but it is a danger we can understand and avoid. As medical researchers scramble to find a cure, it is important to remember that AIDS is preventable. Taking the proper precautions to prevent infection is the first step in fighting this disease that affects so many people in North America and around the world.

There is some good news in the fight against AIDS. The most notable of these is that, thanks to therapies that have been developed over the last decade, many people who are currently infected with HIV live longer, healthier lives than did the first group of people who contracted the virus. Unfortunately, these therapies are costly and are often unavailable to many people across the world, particularly in developing nations. Even in the United States, where annual AIDS-related deaths have declined, the rate of infection is still frighteningly high among minorities and in inner cities. Moreover, many people have become complacent and are again engaging in high-risk behaviors.

There is still a lot of ignorance and misinformation about AIDS in general. It is important to replace these with useful knowledge. In this book, you will learn about HIV/AIDS, its origins, and how it affects the body's immune system. You will also learn how a person contracts HIV, as well as what you can do to protect yourself from becoming infected. Scientists and researchers are working very hard to make this disease extinct. You can play your part by learning how to protect yourself and the people you care about from AIDS transmission and using this knowledge when making choices about your own life.

AIDS DEFINED

HIV is a virus that attacks the body's immune system, making it unable to fight infection. The National Institutes of Health (NIH) defines AIDS as "the most serious stage of HIV infection" that "results from the destruction of the infected person's immune system."[1] The Centers for Disease Control and Prevention (CDC) further explains the disease by defining each word in its name as follows:

---

1 "HIV and Its Treatment: What You Should Know. Health Information for Patients," July 2006. Published by the U.S.Department of Health and Human Services.

Acquired Means that the disease is not hereditary, but develops after birth from contact with a disease-causing agent (in this case, HIV).

Immunodeficiency Means that the disease is characterized by a weakening of the immune system.

Syndrome Refers to a group of symptoms that collectively indicate or characterize a disease. In the case of AIDS, this can include the development of certain infections and/or cancers, as well as a decrease in the number of certain cells in a person's immune system.*

[* Centers for Disease Control and Prevention, "What Is AIDS?" Retrieved June 2006 (http://www.cdc.gov/hiv/resources/qa/qa2.htm).]

A BRIEF HISTORY OF HIV/AIDS

During the late 1970s and early 1980s, doctors became aware that an increasing number of people were suffering from several rare illnesses. One of these illnesses was a respiratory disease, Pneumocystis carinii pneumonia (PCP), which was usually a problem only for cancer patients undergoing chemotherapy. Another was a rare skin cancer, Kaposi's sarcoma, which, until then, mostly affected Mediterranean or Jewish men older than fifty years old who would usually live for years after diagnosis. However, the men becoming ill with these diseases were much younger and had previously been healthy. The diseases progressed so rapidly within their bodies that it appeared as if their immune systems were no longer working to resist them. Consequently, the men became weak and died. The number of cases recognized by doctors in cities across the United States grew from a few dozen in 1980 to several thousand within five years. According to the World Health Organization (WHO), the number of AIDS cases worldwide rose from 2 in 1979 to 185,313 in 1994, for a total of 1,209,997 cases in 1994.*

[* World Health Organization. "Global AIDS Statistics." *Global AIDS Focus AIDS Care,* Vol.8, No.2, pp.246–248. Retrieved August 2006 (http://taylorandfrancis.metapress.com/media/pf9gtmtwxrd97tmxcd4p/contributions/v/6/3/3/v633f8tc0a514087.pdf).]

The Early Victims

At first, very little was known about what was happening. Who was becoming ill? Was this a disease caused by a germ, or was it an immune system illness resulting from drug abuse? Would this condition spread among people at work or school or in cities?

Many of the first few people diagnosed with this condition were homosexual men. Because of this, their condition was referred to as gay-related immunodeficiency, or GRID. However, the condition also showed up in intravenous drug users—male and female—who weren't homosexuals.

Another group of people affected by the so-called gay-related immunodeficiency were hemophiliacs. These people (almost all male) have a rare condition from birth that makes it hard for their blood to clot. They need to have regular injections of a clotting factor derived from blood donations. Many men and youths with hemophilia were ill with this condition, though none of them abused intravenous drugs and few were homosexual. The wives of some infected hemophiliacs also became ill, and that alarmed the medical community even further.

It soon became clear that the illness was contagious, which means that someone could catch it from someone else. It was being passed from the sick men to their sexual partners, both male and female. Another clue lay in the fact that intravenous drug abusers sometimes share needles, which can bring a drop of blood from one person to another. It became obvious that the illness must be caused by something that could be carried in blood. Doctors checked among patients who had received blood transfusions or organ donations and found a few other people who were affected by this new disease.

Solving the Mystery

It took research in hospitals and laboratories all around the world to figure out what was happening: a previously unknown and rare virus had spread from person to person. As people travel from town to town, country to country, and around the world, some carry viruses inside their bodies without knowing it because they do not appear to be ill. Most of these viruses cause the common cold or other diseases that are treatable. But this disease was different. It hadn't been recognized before.

The new disease made a person's immune system stop working so that the person would become ill from multiple causes and die. It was similar in some ways to the immune system weakness suffered by some people being treated for cancer. It was as if a person had acquired the very rare illness of being born with little or no immune system. In 1982, this disease was named acquired immune deficiency syndrome, or acquired immunodeficiency syndrome (AIDS).

Identifying the Culprit

In 1983, the Institut Pasteur in France recognized that a virus was the cause of AIDS. This virus was named human immunodeficiency virus (HIV). Researchers now understood how the virus moved from one person to another by the exchange of semen, blood, or vaginal secretions during sexual contact or by coming into contact with the blood of an infected person, most likely through needle sharing and blood transfusions.

Researchers also learned how HIV weakens the body's immune system by attacking specific white blood cells. White blood cells circulate in the bloodstream and lymph system throughout the body; they are part of the immune system and attack foreign invaders of the body. T-helper cells are the type of white blood cells that help fight off bacteria and viruses that enter the body. HIV attacks and destroys this kind of cell in particular.

Another breakthrough was the achievement in 1985 of a test for HIV antibodies in a person's blood. If a person has HIV, his or her immune system makes antibodies to try to kill the virus. Developing this test was crucial because a person with HIV might not look or feel ill for many months or even years, and may therefore unwittingly pass on the disease to others.

THE ORIGIN OF AIDS

As we've seen, AIDS appeared suddenly, and at first no one knew anything about it. There were rumors based on guesses. Some people wondered if AIDS was caused by an artificial virus that escaped from a research lab. After all, nobody had ever seen a disease like this before. Did it come from outer space on a meteor? Others worried that maybe AIDS was a weapon invented to kill certain people. These rumors are not true. HIV was not invented by scientists. It was not created in a modern laboratory. It did not come from outer space on a meteor or a spaceship.

HIV is a natural virus that used to be very rare and once affected only a few types of monkeys and chimpanzees in Africa. It is related to simian immunodeficiency virus, a similar immune deficiency virus that affects monkeys and apes (simians). People were exposed to HIV when they caught the monkeys for food or kept them as pets. Perhaps by being scratched or bitten, these people were exposed to the virus in the monkey blood.

There are a few human blood samples more than fifty years old that test positive for HIV. It is believed that the first human infections with HIV might have occurred between 1930 and 1950.

A POSITIVE OUTLOOK

It can be depressing and discouraging to realize that even modern medicine cannot eliminate a disease from the world. The only disease that has been completely eliminated is smallpox. Even so, there are still frozen samples of the smallpox virus kept securely in a few research laboratories. A virus such as HIV is much harder to recognize than smallpox; unlike smallpox victims, a person who carries HIV may not look or feel sick for many months or years. By the time a person is diagnosed with AIDS, it may not be possible for him or her to find everyone whom he or she may have accidentally infected with HIV.

But the news is not all bad. People have always had to live with diseases and illnesses of many kinds. In the past, and still today in some parts of the world, ignorance meant that sick people were shunned or blamed for their illness. There used to be no useful treatment for many kinds of illness. Some treatments used to be available only at great cost, for the wealthy. People used to suffer and die from simple illnesses that can now be treated with modern medicine and good nutrition.

There are many things that can help a person with HIV or AIDS to live well, from medicine to eating well, exercising, and getting rest. The support of family and friends is also a big help.

There is plenty of good news about living in a world where HIV exists. HIV is not as easy to catch as a cold or the flu, or hepatitis, tuberculosis, or polio. All of those diseases can sometimes be passed from one person to another by shaking hands, sharing food, or breathing on each other. HIV is a much more delicate virus. It is not airborne. It does not live outside of a human body. When it gets cold or dries up, HIV dies.

Although HIV can pass from one person to another during sex, there are ways to make infection much less likely. The same safe-sex methods that make it less likely to pass on HIV also prevent the sharing of some other sexually transmitted diseases.

CHAPTER TWO

Contracting the Virus

THE GENDER OF THE PEOPLE TOUCHING DOES NOT MATTER. THE VIRUS CAN BE TRANSMITTED FROM A MAN TO A WOMAN, FROM A WOMAN TO A MAN, FROM A MAN TO A MAN, AND FROM A WOMAN TO A WOMAN.

Because many of the first people to be diagnosed with AIDS were homosexual men, there were rumors at first that only gay men ever got this disease. These rumors have been proved to be wrong. HIV is spread from person to person primarily by sexual contact that involves an exchange of body fluids. According to the CDC, 80 percent of all HIV/AIDS cases diagnosed in the United States in 2004 were the result of sexual contact.[2]

The gender of the people touching does not matter. The virus can be transmitted from a man to a woman, from a woman to a man, from a man to a man, or from a woman to a woman. Nevertheless, males account for 73 percent of American adults and adoles-

---

2 The Centers for Disease Control and Prevention, HIV/AIDS Surveillance Report: Cases of HIV Infection and AIDS in the United States, 2004.

cents living with HIV/AIDS.[3] If a man who has HIV does not wear a condom, the virus in his semen and pre-seminal fluid could infect his partner. A woman who has HIV could infect her partner with the virus from her vaginal fluids. Any tiny cut or sore inside a vagina, anus, or mouth or on a penis would make it easy for the virus to pass into a person's body. A tiny sore like this is usually too small to see or feel.

HIV is also transmitted by coming into contact with an infected person's blood, most likely by sharing needles during injection drug use. Close to 20 percent of all Americans living with HIV/AIDS were infected this way.[4] A pregnant woman who is HIV positive can also pass the virus to her unborn child. While the incidence of children being born with HIV is only fractional in the United States, the rates are significantly higher in other parts of the world where anti-HIV therapies are not as readily available.

---

3 Ibid.

4 "HIV and Its Treatment: What You Should Know. Health Information for Patients," July2006. Published by the U.S. Department of Health and Human Services.

WHY HEMOPHILIACS ARE VULNERABLE

Hemophiliacs need regular injections of a blood-clotting product (made from the blood cells of others) all their lives. Consequently, they are more vulnerable to the risk of a blood-carried disease. Most people might need only a single transfusion in their lifetimes because of surgery or an accident, and might need only one unit of blood donated by one generous person. But hemophiliacs need a blood product made by pooling several blood donations and sorting out the clotting factor and other parts for many uses. If one blood donor is HIV positive, many hemophiliacs could be infected.

Since 1986, every time people donate blood, they are questioned carefully about whether they have done anything that puts them at risk of HIV infection. And every unit of blood is tested for HIV antibodies. This is true everywhere in North America and Europe, and most countries in the world try to meet this standard as well.

NO INFECTIONS FROM INSECT BITES

For many years, people feared coming into contact with HIV-infected persons because they didn't understand how the disease was transmitted. Also, because HIV operates in blood, the fear of infection through insect bites seemed reasonable for a while. However, HIV transmission mainly takes place through a number of high-risk behaviors, namely unprotected sex and needle sharing.

Insects that bite humans, like mosquitoes, ticks, or bedbugs, can take a tiny drop of blood from a person. But HIV cannot survive inside these insects because the virus is too frail. Even if an insect bites a person who is HIV positive or has AIDS, the insect will not get infected and it cannot infect another person. There are other diseases carried by insect bites, but not AIDS, since HIV cannot be transmitted by insect bites. The following are a number of situations that will not lead to an HIV infection:

- Touching a doorknob that has been touched by a person who is HIV positive
- Being friends with or working with a person who is HIV positive
- Touching a toilet seat that has been used by a person who is HIV positive
- Donating blood

- Swimming in a pool with a person who is HIV positive
- Sharing food or a drink with an HIV-positive person, or even drinking from the same straw
- Kissing

THE GENETICS OF HIV

Like other viruses, HIV cannot grow or reproduce on its own. A virus must infect the cells of a living organism—a person, an animal, or a plant—in order to make new copies of itself.

HIV is one of a special class of virus called retroviruses. A retrovirus uses a reverse version of some standard enzymes in our cells. Almost all organisms, including most viruses, store their genetic material on long molecules of DNA (deoxyribonucleic acid). But the genes of retro-viruses are made of RNA (ribonucleic acid). RNA has a very similar structure to DNA.

HIV has just nine genes. That's not many compared to the more than 500 genes in some bacteria, or around 20,000 to 25,000 genes in a human. These genes can mutate, making tiny changes in the virus.

INSIDE HUMAN CELLS

When a virus gets inside a living cell, it uses the cell's own copying process to make copies of itself as well. When this copying process is hijacked by a lethal virus such as HIV, the result is a lot of copies of the virus and a dead cell.

HIV uses chemicals called enzymes to get into a cell, hide itself there, and get copies of itself made. Once inside a human cell, HIV uses an enzyme, reverse transcriptase, to convert its own viral RNA into DNA. In the cell's nucleus, this DNA is spliced into the human DNA by another HIV enzyme, called integrate. That integrated HIV DNA may remain dormant within a cell for a long time.

But when the cell becomes activated to make new proteins for many uses, it treats the HIV genes much like human genes. First, the cell uses human enzymes to convert the genes into messenger RNA, then the RNA is transported outside the nucleus to be a blueprint for producing new proteins and enzymes. Some of these RNA strands are complete copies of HIV, which are released from the cell in particles ready to infect other cells. Unlike most bacteria, HIV particles are too small to be seen with an ordinary microscope.

This process may seem very complicated. The most practical part to know is that the enzymes used to convert or copy the virus are able to be slowed down, or inhibited, by certain drugs prescribed by doctors.

SYMPTOMS

A person who is HIV positive can live for years without developing any symptoms. But there are some common warning signs of HIV infection. If you suffer from one of these common warning signs, do not be alarmed. It does not mean that you have HIV. Many other illnesses have similar symptoms. The symptoms of HIV infection are not unique, they just show that a person's immune system is being stressed. It's up to a doctor to diagnose the illness that is causing the symptoms.

Swollen lymph nodes are early warning signs of HIV infection. Lymph nodes are part of the immune system. They are small, bean-shaped organs that are also called glands. You can sometimes feel them in your neck, armpits, and groin. Other nodes are deep inside the body. Lymph nodes store immune cells, which can trap and destroy bacteria and viruses that enter the body. A lymph node swells as the immune cells inside the node attack foreign invaders.

Other possible warning signs of HIV infection include a flu-like illness (usually experienced within weeks after exposure to HIV), frequent fevers, excessive sweating, unexplained fatigue, rapid weight loss, pneumonia, breathing difficulties, or diarrhea that lasts longer than a week. A person with HIV could develop white spots or sores in the mouth and throat, or blotches on or under the skin that are colored red, pink, purple, or brown.

DIAGNOSING HIV AND AIDS

It takes a doctor's diagnosis to recognize who has HIV or AIDS. This is done with a simple blood test. A person who has been infected with HIV will test positive for the antibody. Such a person is said to be HIV positive. We cannot diagnose ourselves just by how we look or feel.

People whose infections have progressed to AIDS may be recognized by the diseases from which they are suffering. Because their immune systems are no longer working, people with AIDS are vulnerable to close to twenty illnesses, called AIDS-defining conditions. The list, as published by the Centers for Disease Control and Prevention in 1992, includes:

- Candidiasis

- Cervical cancer (invasive)
- Coccidioidomycosis, cryptococcosis, cryptosporidiosis
- Cytomegalovirus disease
- Encephalopathy (HIV-related)
- Herpes simplex (severe infection)
- Histoplasmosis
- Isosporiasis
- Kaposi's sarcoma
- Lymphoma (certain types)
- Mycobacterium avium complex
- Pneumocystis carinii/jiroveci pneumonia
- Pneumonia (recurrent)
- Progressive multifocal leukoencephalopathy
- Salmonella septicemia (recurrent)
- Toxoplasmosis of the brain

- Tuberculosis
- Wasting syndrome*

[* The Centers for Disease Control and Prevention, "Living with HIV/AIDS." Updated September 2005. (http://www.cdc.gov/hiv/pubs/brochure/livingwithhiv.htm).]

It is important to note that many people suffer from these conditions without having AIDS. To be diagnosed with AIDS, a person must first be infected with HIV. Doctors carefully observe and count the white blood cells of HIV patients. There are normally tens of thousands of white blood cells in a healthy body. When the T-helper cell count (also referred to as the CD4 count) drops below 200, a person is formally diagnosed with AIDS. It may also be diagnosed even if the HIV-positive patient's CD4 count is more than 200 and he or she has one or more of the AIDS-defining conditions.[5]

STAGES OF HIV AND AIDS

The Centers for Disease Control and Prevention (CDC) recognizes several steps in the progression from HIV infection to AIDS. They are:

---

5 Ibid.

- **Infection:** The earliest stage is right after you are infected. HIV can infect cells and copy itself before your immune system has started to respond. You may have felt flulike symptoms during this time.

- **Response:** The next stage is when your body responds to the virus. Even if you don't feel any different, your body is trying to fight the virus by making antibodies against it. This is called seroconversion, when you go from being HIV negative to HIV positive.

- **No symptoms:** You may enter a stage in which you have no symptoms. This is called asymptomatic infection. You still have HIV, and it may be causing damage that you can't feel.

- **Symptoms:** Symptomatic HIV infection is when you develop symptoms such as certain infections, including Pneumocystis carinii pneumonia.

- **AIDS:** AIDS is diagnosed when you have a variety of symptoms, infections, and specific test results. There is no single test to diagnose AIDS.[6]

---

6 The Centers for Disease Control and Prevention, HIV/AIDS Surveillance Report: Cases of HIV Infection and AIDS in the United States, 2004.

Although a person may show no visible signs or symptoms during the asymptomatic stage, the virus is reproducing more than 10 billion copies of itself per day inside the body. The symptomatic stage may be subdivided into two periods: the early symptomatic stage and the late symptomatic stage. During the early symptomatic stage, an infected person begins to show symptoms such as fever, night sweats, fatigue, weight loss, swollen lymph nodes, diarrhea, breathing difficulties, or vision problems. The late symptomatic stage begins when the immune system of the infected person begins to weaken. The early symptoms may continue or become more frequent, and new symptoms will begin. These may include cancer, shingles (a disease of the skin), and extreme weight loss from AIDS wasting syndrome. The benchmark for defining AIDS continues to change as medical research unveils new ways of treating and controlling the disease. However, generally, the most defining statistic is a T-cell count below 200, coupled with the presence of one or more AIDS-defining conditions, which are also known as opportunistic infections.

THE LATER STAGES

People who have AIDS are at a higher risk of suffering from certain mental disorders. Memory loss is one of the disorders, and another is dementia, a severe loss of mental capacity. Another common brain disorder causes many AIDS patients to lose feeling in their arms and legs.

AIDS-related cancers include Kaposi's sarcoma (KS), which causes purplish marks called lesions on the skin, the linings of the digestive tract, and the lungs. KS was rare before the 1980s, but now most cases of KS occur in people with AIDS. Lymphoma is cancer of the white blood cells (lymphocytes). People with advanced HIV infection have a higher-than-average risk of developing lymphoma. Women who are HIV positive have an increased risk of developing cervical cancer. There are no symptoms associated with the early stages of this cancer, but there is a test for the early cell changes, called a Pap test, which should be taken yearly by women.

LIFE EXPECTANCY

Some people progress quickly from infection with HIV to showing symptoms after only a few months; they may die within two years, usually from an illness that takes advantage of the immune system failure. This is more common where there is little medical care, in developing countries, but it can happen anywhere.

In North America, where medical care is available and people usually enjoy good health and nutrition, the news is somewhat better. Some people stay asymptomatic for many months and even years. Others stay at the early symptomatic stage for many months or years. In 2004, the CDC found that only 39 percent of Americans diagnosed as HIV positive in 2003 received an AIDS diagnosis in fewer than twelve months. For a while, once a person was diagnosed with AIDS, he or she usually lived for less than two years. However, the CDC also found that among Americans diagnosed with AIDS after 2000, 90 percent survived for more than a year, 86 percent survived for more than two years, and 83 percent survived for more than three years.[7] The main reason for these amazing survival rates is the development of retroviral drugs over the last decade.

---

7 Ibid

CHAPTER THREE

Prevention

ABSTINENCE, NOT HAVING SEXUAL INTERCOURSE, IS THE ONLY SURE WAY TO AVOID CONTRACTING HIV BY SEXUAL CONTACT. HOWEVER, IF YOU'RE GOING TO HAVE SEX, THEN IT IS IMPORTANT TO PRACTICE SAFE SEX.

AIDS is not a disease that gets better and goes away. It cannot be cured by medicine or beliefs or clean living. The only defense against AIDS and HIV is prevention. HIV is not an unavoidable disaster like an earthquake; it is just a virus that lives inside human bodies. The only way to prevent the spread of AIDS is to avoid the behaviors that transmit HIV from person to person. Chief among these are unprotected sex and intravenous drug use.

UNPROTECTED SEX IS HIGH-RISK BEHAVIOR

HIV is most commonly spread by body fluids—blood, semen, and vaginal fluids—during sexual contact. It can be passed sexually from male to female, from male to male, from female to male, and rarely from female to female. The virus is most likely to be transmitted by contacting body fluids with an open sore or a break in the skin.

Sexual contact includes anything involving a penis, vagina, anus, or mouth. Most methods of safe sex involve using a condom or dental dam as a barrier, to prevent contact with body fluids. Unprotected sexual contact means that no barrier is used. Even the first time a person has sex, it's important to have protected sex. (There is no truth to the myth that having sex with a virgin can cure AIDS.) Also, the more sexual partners that a person has, the more likely it is that he or she will have sex with someone who is HIV positive. Even if both partners are HIV positive, they should still have protected sex, to avoid being infected with different versions of HIV.

SAFE SEX IS LOWER-RISK BEHAVIOR

Abstinence, not having sexual intercourse, is the only sure way to avoid contracting HIV by sexual contact. However, if you're going to have sex, then it is important to practice safe sex. Sexual touching does not have to be high-risk behavior. Kissing, touching with hands, and rubbing bodies will not transmit HIV from one person to another. Masturbating by yourself or with someone watching will not transmit HIV.

Intercourse is much less likely to transmit the virus if a barrier is used. A barrier is usually a latex condom or dental dam. Avoid condoms that are made from animal membranes because germs can get through them. A lubricating cream or jelly should also be used, one that kills HIV and is spermicidal (kills sperm). This will make the barrier less likely to break, and if the barrier does break, the lubricant will be there to kill sperm or the virus. The lubricant should be a water-based brand. It is unsafe to use Vaseline, baby oil, and cooking oil as lubricants because these may cause the condom to break.

AVERT, a UK-based international HIV and AIDS charity, advises against the use of condoms and lubricants that contain a spermicide called Nonoxynol-9, which was once thought to help prevent the spread of HIV, but has since been proved ineffective. According to AVERT, "Some people have an allergic reaction to Nonoxynol-9 that can result in little sores, which can actually make the transmission of HIV more likely. Because of this, you should only use condoms and lubricants containing Nonoxynol-9 if you are HIV negative and know that your partner is, too. Nevertheless, using a condom (even if it contains Nonoxynol-9) is much safer than having unprotected sex."*

[* "Using Condoms, Condom Types & Condom Sizes." Avert.com. Retrieved August 2006 (http://www.avert.org/usecond.htm).]

A man should put a latex condom on his penis before touching a partner's vagina, mouth, anus, or penis. Anything that enters a person's vagina, mouth, or anus should be covered with a condom. Partners should not share sex toys with each other or with anyone else.

A woman should use lubricant if her male partner is using a condom. A woman could also use a lubricant and a female condom to line her vagina if her male partner is not using a condom. If a woman is using the birth control pill, her male partner should use a condom as well, as the pill offers no protection against sexually transmitted diseases.

If a woman is using a diaphragm or cervical cap or sponge for birth control, even with lubricant this is not enough protection for safe sex. These methods of birth control block sperm from entering a woman's uterus, but they would not block HIV from entering tiny sores inside her vagina. They are helpful at reducing the risk of HIV infection, but they do not provide sufficient protection. Therefore, it is essential that her male partner use a condom as well.

A person who is allowing a penis or finger or anything else to enter her or his anus should use lubricant, as the anus is very easily damaged. Any tiny sores would allow HIV into the body.

A dental dam is a sheet of latex that can be used between a woman's vagina and a person's mouth, or between an anus and a mouth. If you can't find dental dams at a store, you can make one by unrolling a condom and cutting it open along one side to make a flat sheet of latex. Although the lubricant may not taste very good, it is safe to get in the mouth during sex. Latex gloves are another option—a glove can be used to cover fingers or a sex toy, and another glove can be cut open to make a flat sheet of latex for a dental dam.

Judy was walking hand in hand with Eric after a meal at the only place in town you could get a takeout hamburger. It wasn't far to his place from here, and she was looking forward to spending the rest of the evening together. Most of the businesses along the road were already closed when he stopped at the drugstore.

"Do you want some gum, or chips, or something?" Eric asked. "I need to go get some condoms before we make love."

"No, you don't have to bother with those anymore." Judy tugged his hand so he'd move a little closer and said quietly, "Don't worry about me getting pregnant. I'm on the pill

now." She was glad it was getting dark. Maybe he wouldn't see that she was blushing.

"We should still use condoms, too, so we don't have to worry about AIDS," he said.

"Why would we worry about that?" Judy shrugged. "This isn't the big city. I don't have it. You don't have it. Nobody around here would have AIDS."

"Well, I know someone here who lived in Los Angeles for a while before moving here, and someone else who visited Toronto. Those are pretty big cities."

"Do you figure I might have slept with them? How many people do you think..."

"No, I don't mean that!" he said quickly. "I just meant it's not a big city thing. It's about treating you right. I want to make this safe for you. It's up to me to use a condom. If you can take the pill, I should do my part, too."

"Yeah, I get it. That's, like, being together on this." Judy smiled and squeezed his hand. "It's kind of sweet, you wanting to be so responsible."

"That's just the kind of guy I am."

PREGNANCY AND VERTICAL TRANSMISSION OF HIV

Of course, a common consequence of unprotected sex is an unwanted pregnancy, particularly among teens. According to the National Campaign to Prevent Teen Pregnancy, 34 percent of young women become pregnant at least once before they are twenty years old. Of these, 81 percent are unintended pregnancies and 80 percent are to unmarried teens.*

[* The National Campaign to Prevent Teen Pregnancy, "General Facts and Stats." Teenpregnancy.org. Retrieved August 2006 (http://www.teenpregnancy.org/resources/data/genlfact.asp).]

HIV can also be transmitted from a pregnant mother to her unborn child, or from a nursing mother to her child in her milk. This is sometimes called vertical transmission. There are medications to reduce the risk of passing the virus to the unborn child to 1 chance in 4. Fortunately, the incidence of HIV and AIDS among newborn infants has declined significantly in the United States over the years, with an estimated total of 48 in 2004.* Moreover, many women who are HIV positive think that risk is too high and have decided not to become pregnant.

[* "United States HIV & AIDS Statistics Summary." Avert.com. Retrieved August 2006 (http://www.avert.org/statsum.htm).]

FIDELITY IS LOW-RISK BEHAVIOR

For some people, the preferred option for low-risk behavior is fidelity—both partners choose to have sex only with each other. One of the best reasons for not having sex outside of marriage or other committed relationships is being sure that each partner will not bring an HIV infection—or other disease—to the other. As for being sure about your partner, this behavior choice relies on trust and keeping promises.

SOME THINGS THAT DO NOT SPREAD HIV

Research has shown that some body fluids do not transmit HIV to another person, even though the fluids come from someone who is HIV positive. These body fluids have substances or chemicals in them naturally that stop the virus from being infectious (able to infect anyone). Body fluids that do not transmit HIV from an infected person include tears, saliva, sweat, urine, and feces.

Research has also proved that we do not have to be afraid of transmitting HIV from one person to another by shaking hands or holding hands, hugging, or kissing, or even coughing and sneezing. HIV cannot be spread by living in the same house or sharing household objects as a person who is HIV positive. You can use a public swimming pool or a public toilet, or go to work or school without worrying about whether anyone else there is HIV positive.

Prolonged Kissing

Though there is some HIV in the saliva of people who are HIV positive, saliva contains substances that stop HIV from being infectious. There is no evidence that the virus is ever spread through saliva. Closed-mouth kissing (dry kissing or social kissing) with an infected person is considered safe. In the case of open-mouth kissing (French kissing), it would be better to be cautious if either partner has sores or wounds in or around the mouth.

SHARING NEEDLES IS HIGH-RISK BEHAVIOR

HIV can be spread when people who abuse intravenous drugs share needles. As noted before, roughly 20 percent of all HIV infections are caused this way. But that's only half of the picture. According to the CDC, "Injection drug use contributes to the epidemic's spread far beyond the circle of those who inject. People who have sex with an injection drug user

(IDU) also are at risk for an infection through the sexual transmission of HIV. Children born to mothers who contracted HIV through sharing needles or having sex with an IDU may become infected as well." The CDC estimates that, to date, injection drug use has directly or indirectly contributed to about 36 percent of AIDS cases in the United States.* Other diseases such as hepatitis C can be transmitted this way, too. Moreover, injecting illegal drugs is generally unsafe and hazardous to your health. Among other things, you risk a deadly overdose.

[* Centers for Disease Control and Prevention, "Drug-Associated HIV Transmission Continues in the United States," May 2002. Retrieved August 2006 (http://www.cdc.gov/hiv/resources/factsheets/idu.htm).]

People can avoid this risk of AIDS completely by not using injection drugs. However, for those who cannot or will not stop using drugs, it is important that they not share needles and syringes or use them more than once. There are many programs that help drug abusers quit using drugs and/or provide clean needles.

The CDC also notes that the abuse of noninjection drugs also contributes to the spread of AIDS. In one study of 2,000 young adults in three inner-city neighborhoods, the agency found that smokers of crack cocaine were three times more likely to be infected with HIV than non-smokers.[8] People often make bad decisions, including engaging in risky sexual behaviors, when they are high.

GETTING A TATTOO OR PIERCING

Everyone who gets a tattoo or a piercing is trusting the person who holds the needle. Can you trust this person? Was he or she trained and certified by a public health authority? The fact is, if you are tattooed or pierced with a needle that was previously used on a person who is HIV positive, you could be given the virus. Professional tattoo and piercing studios have machines that will sterilize their equipment, and the person who does the piercing or tattoo should be trained properly and use only new, sterile needles for each person. Ask questions about what methods will be used. And if you do decide to get a tattoo or piercing, have an HIV test a couple months afterward because getting a tattoo or piercing is considered a high-risk behavior.

Chris was sitting on the floor, drawing in his notebook when his mother came home. "Hi, Mom, how was work?"

---

8 Ibid.

"Pretty good today, but I've got to get off my feet. Just a few minutes and I'll make dinner." His mom sat on the couch and looked over at his notebook. "What are you drawing?"

"I'm working on a design for a tattoo I want to have."

"You are not getting any tattoos, young man."

Chris held the notebook up for her to see better. "I've been thinking about this image for a long time, since we went to that museum by the lake. Remember?"

"I remember," said his mom. "The design does look really nice. But that wouldn't make up for putting germs in your body in some filthy back room. You are not tattooing yourself."

"I wouldn't go to some dirty place," Chris protested. "And I wouldn't do it myself. I'd get a real tattoo artist to do a good job."

"They're not all professionals like dentists. I don't know how to find one who is trained to be clean and..." His mother sighed. "What if you got AIDS from a dirty needle? Or hepatitis? I worry about things like that, Chris."

Chris thought his mom sometimes worried too much. "Would you worry as much if I got my ear pierced instead?"

"Oh, no. Now I have to worry about infected earlobes?"

"Aunt Ann's ears are pierced, and they don't get infected," he pointed out.

"You know, you're right," his mom said. "And she's a nurse. You ask Aunt Ann where you might get your ear pierced properly, how to keep it clean, and all. Then come tell me and we'll go together."

"That sounds pretty good." Chris thought of something else. "Aunt Ann might know how to find a good tattoo artist, so you wouldn't worry about me getting AIDS or anything. We could do research."

"It would take a lot of research to change my mind," said his mom. "That will take time. Don't rush." She stood up slowly. "For now, let's start making dinner."

VISITING THE DOCTOR OR DENTIST

Doctors and nurses around the world work to keep medical procedures such as injections or blood transfusions from spreading HIV. Because of education among health care workers, blood products are tested carefully, equipment and instruments are sterilized, and the chances of anyone being infected with HIV are very small.

In North America, doctors, dentists, and their assistants are all trained in how to avoid transmitting HIV from one person to another. New needles are used for each patient, for example, and used needles are discarded safely. When treating a patient with HIV, your doctor or dentist will take special precautions before, during, and after treatment. If you are HIV positive, it is essential to inform your doctor and dentist. The chances that anyone could get HIV from visiting a doctor's or dentist's office are extremely small.

In other countries around the world, the standards of health care may vary. Most health care providers are very careful to protect their patients and themselves.

AVOIDING HIGH-RISK BEHAVIOR

It can be difficult to say no to sex or drug use, but avoiding these two behaviors is how we can protect ourselves and each other from disease. Your decisions should be respected by your friends, boyfriend or girlfriend, and family. You have the right to protect your life—and the lives of people you care about—by saying no.

No one has the right to make you do anything sexually that you don't want to, especially anything that makes you feel uncomfortable or puts you at risk. No one has the right to insist you use illegal drugs in dangerous ways.

How can you respond to pressure about sex or drugs? There are some things you can say:

- "I care about you, but I don't want to have sex."
- "I care about you, but I don't want to have sex until I'm married."
- "I'm not ready, and since this is my body, I'll tell you when I am ready."
- "I'm not ready right now. Let's make a plan for how we'll be safe when we do have sex."

- "I am very sure. You heard me say no, and I mean it."

- "I'm taking care of my body, and I don't want to harm it with drugs."

- "Drugs are illegal, and I will not break the law."

You can probably think of more things to say that would work better for the people you know. Just glaring and frowning and walking away without saying anything can express your feelings pretty clearly, too.

If you should decide to have sex, be smart about it. You cannot tell whether your partner might have HIV. In many cases, he or she might not know either. Unprotected sex is risky. Using latex condoms means that HIV has fewer chances of being transmitted during sexual contact. Use condoms during any sexual activity, meaning vaginal, anal, and oral sex.

EDUCATION CAN HELP

We can learn not to spread this disease. We can each learn about AIDS and HIV. Even people who choose not to have sex can choose to know what are low-risk and high-risk behaviors.

There are programs that teach drug abusers how to clean needles, and even some that hand out clean needles as well as give advice on how to quit drugs. These programs are controversial, though, since some people object to health care programs spending any money on drug abusers. But education can help anyone make better health choices, and it is cheaper than hospital care. Education reduces the spread of disease among drug abusers and their families.

Some parents worry that if their children talk about sex at all, the children will have sex at a very young age, outside of marriage, and with many different partners. But research shows that this is not so. Education helps many young people decide to wait before having sex and to make responsible choices when they do. "Research studies investigating the impact of sexual health education on adolescent behavior consistently find that providing sexual health education does not lead to earlier or more frequent sexual activity," wrote D. Kirby, in an article for the *Handbook of HIV Prevention.*[9]

---

9 D. Kirby, "School-Based Interventions to Prevent Unprotected Sex and HIV Among Adolescents," Handbook of HIV Prevention. J. Peterson and R. Diclemente, eds. (New York, NY: Plenum Publishers, 2000).

CHAPTER FOUR

Getting Tested

EVERYONE SHOULD KNOW HIS OR HER HIV STATUS, ESPECIALLY THOSE PEOPLE WHO ENGAGE IN OR HAVE ENGAGED IN ANY HIGH-RISK BEHAVIOR.

Although there is no cure for AIDS, it is important that people become aware of what it is and how to avoid contracting HIV. Everyone should know his or her HIV status, especially those people who engage in or have engaged in any high-risk behavior. There's no need to wonder or worry if you might be HIV positive—get tested and you'll know for sure. The test for HIV antibodies is very reliable and is available throughout North America.

According to the CDC, approximately 25 percent of Americans who are infected with HIV do not know that they are infected.* Research also shows that most people who know that they are infected take steps to reduce their risk of infecting others. Given these two realities, it makes sense that increasing the number of people who know their HIV status can help to reduce HIV transmission. More important, more HIV-positive individuals would get the treatment they need. Accordingly, the CDC is recommending that HIV testing become part of routine medical examinations.** Ultimately, it is every person's responsibility to find out his or her HIV status.

[* Centers for Disease Control and Prevention, "HIV/AIDS Among Men Who Have Sex with Men." Retrieved July 2006 (http://www.cdc.gov/hiv/resources/factsheets/msm.htm).]

[** Daniel DeNoon, "CDC: Everyone to Get HIV Test." WebMD. Retrieved August 2006 (http://www.webmd.com/content/article/121/114438.htm).]

THE TESTS

It's very easy to get tested for HIV. A small amount of blood is drawn from your arm by a doctor, nurse, or clinic worker using a sterilized syringe. This blood test takes only a few minutes, and you'll just feel a small poke with the needle.

The blood is then sent to a laboratory to be tested. The results will be made known to you after one to three weeks. There are different places you can go to get tested, and the test can be done anonymously or confidentially.

PLACES FOR TESTING

You can choose one of many places to go for an HIV test. Hospitals, clinics, private doctor's offices, family planning or sexually transmitted disease clinics, health departments, and mobile sites offer HIV testing. Some of these places charge for an HIV test, while others offer it for free.

There is a list of resources in the Where to Go for Help section at the back of this book. These organizations can direct you to resources that are available in your community. After you decide where you want to be tested, you can choose whether you prefer an anonymous test or a confidential test.

ANONYMOUS HIV TESTING

If you take an anonymous HIV test, you do not have to give your name. A unique code will be used to identify you instead. The only person who will know your actual test results is you. This type of test is available in most states.

You can also use an at-home test, or collection kit, to be anonymous. This test can be ordered over the phone or the Internet, and it will be shipped to you. You have to take a sample of your own blood, as explained in the kit, and then send it to a laboratory. The test results will be sent to you in a few weeks.

The results are not given to anyone else, and most are considered to be quite accurate.

Notwithstanding the convenience of the home tests, most HIV experts would advise people to have their HIV tests done in a medical setting, where counseling (both before and after the test) is a part of the testing process. Most people dread the thought of being HIV positive and are therefore extremely anxious about taking the test. Counseling helps to allay these anxieties, particularly if the result comes back positive.

CONFIDENTIAL HIV TESTING

Confidential HIV testing is also called names testing. Unlike anonymous HIV testing, you are required to give your name, and the result is released only to the medical personnel who administered the test and, in some states, the state health department. Also, you can choose to have the result added to your medical record. All states make this type of HIV test available.

> *"Toya, instead of catching the bus, can I walk you home today?" asked Martin.*
>
> *"Sure," said Toya. "It's pretty far, though."*
>
> *"I'll carry your backpack," he said and took it. "I want to ask you something."*

"OK, what is it?"

Martin walked along without talking for a while before asking, "Do you know if that clinic on Thursdays, in that green building, is just for girls to get the birth control pill, or do they do AIDS tests there, too?"

"I heard they do tests for HIV, which causes AIDS. Martin, what have you done?"

He shook his head. "I don't want to talk about that. I just want to know if I could go there for a test. Nah, it probably doesn't matter. Just forget it."

"I can't just forget it!" Toya protested. "You're my friend. You should have a test for HIV."

"I don't want anyone to recognize me going in there." He tried to laugh. "They'll know I'm not going in for a prescription for birth control pills."

Toya gave him a friendly shove. "Yeah, right. Well, there's another clinic I heard about over on Cook Street on Wednesday nights. We could go there."

"We? Hey, I don't need someone to hold my hand," said Martin. "I'll go there sometime by myself."

"Well, I'll get tested, too."

"You?" Martin couldn't believe it. "You'd never worry about AIDS. You never use drugs. And you told me you never had sex with anyone."

"Not the kind of sex that, you know, could make babies," Toya said. "But TJ and I, we ... um..."

"Oh," said Martin. "Did you have oral sex? Can people catch AIDS from that?"

"It's not a high risk. But I should have an HIV test so I know for sure. I should have thought about it then," she admitted. "But I can think about it now."

"OK, then we'll both go on Wednesday to get tested." Martin laughed. "But in the meantime, I'm going to try not to think about it."

RESPONSIBILITY

Being tested for HIV is a way to take responsibility for your own life and actions. It's a smart choice that helps you take control of your health care. It can be scary to wait for test results and the potential consequences, but knowing the truth can help you make good choices.

THE TEST ITSELF IS NO RISK

Are you hesitating to get your blood tested for HIV because you're worried that the needle used could possibly infect you? Or maybe you're hesitating about donating blood. You do not have to worry about this at all. There is no risk at all of HIV or AIDS from having your blood tested or from donating blood. In Canada and the United States, all doctors, nurses, and blood technicians always use a brand-new, sterile needle for each person. No needles are ever reused on someone else. No one else's blood will ever be put into your body when a sample of your blood is taken or when you donate blood. You can have complete confidence.

CHAPTER FIVE

Dealing with an HIV-Positive Diagnosis

THERE IS AN INCREDIBLE NETWORK OF SUPPORT ORGANIZATIONS ACROSS THE UNITED STATES THAT IS EAGER TO OFFER AID, INFORMATION, AND COMFORT TO HIV-POSITIVE INDIVIDUALS.

For most people, learning that you are HIV positive may be the most devastating news that you can receive. However, it is important to realize that, unlike when it was first discovered, HIV is not a death sentence. Many people, including basketball great Magic Johnson, go on to live long, productive lives after they discover their HIV-positive status. You can, too.

A positive HIV test doesn't mean you have AIDS. However, HIV can progress to AIDS if it remains untreated. Therefore, some of the first things you should do after learning your status is to find out more about the disease, seek support, and see an HIV doctor. Chances are that if you did your HIV test in a medical setting, the doctor, nurse, or a counselor there would have given you some information about how to go about doing these things.

TELLING A LOVED ONE

Many people recall feeling terribly alone when they first tested positive for HIV. Although this is a normal reaction, it is important to recognize that there is an incredible network of support organizations across the United States that is eager to offer aid, information, and comfort to HIV-positive individuals. However, no matter how willing these groups are to help, they recognize the importance of being able to share your diagnosis with someone you trust, especially if that person is a loved one. "Connecting with others ... while you're adjusting to the news is one of the 'first steps' we recommend," says Regan Hofmann, editor-in-chief of *POZ* magazine.[10]

Ideally, teenagers who test positive for HIV without their parents' knowledge should inform their parents right away. No matter how disappointed or upset you think your parents may become, it is generally unwise to keep such a critical diagnosis from the very people who are most responsible for your well-being.

Enlist the help of someone else, like a counselor from the clinic where you did the test, to break the news to your parents if you feel you cannot face them alone. You're likely to find that your parents will rally

---

10 Regan Hofmann, "The Same Old Me." POZ, November 2005, p.3.

to your support no matter how shocked they are by the news. If, however, your parents are not supportive, choose someone else whom you think will be able to handle the news and keep your secret. Although it is difficult to tell how people will respond, you should have an idea of who will be there for you.

Regardless of the support you get from your family, you should consider joining a support group for people who are recently diagnosed with HIV. (There are support groups for parents of HIV-positive people, too.) Such groups can be instrumental for easing your anxieties, providing you with reliable information, and steering you in the right direction for the various services, including medical treatment, that you might need.

FINDING A DOCTOR

It is important to see an HIV doctor as soon as possible after receiving an HIV-positive diagnosis. The initial test determines only your HIV status; you'll need to undergo further tests to find out how the virus is affecting your body and how soon you'll need treatment. HIV care is ongoing. Unless a cure is found, you'll likely be seeing your doctor every three or four months for the rest of your life. Therefore, it is important that you find the right doctor for you.

Finding a doctor is not difficult. Your current primary care doctor may be an HIV specialist, or he or she may be able to refer you to one. You may also seek the advice of other HIV-positive people, a support group, AIDS services organizations, or even the clinic or medical center where you did the test.

Some people interview several doctors before signing on as a patient. However you go about selecting your HIV specialist, here are a few questions you should keep in mind in deciding who is right for you:

- Does the doctor have experience dealing with HIV?
- Does the doctor make you feel comfortable?
- Did the doctor answer your questions clearly?
- Is the doctor available enough?
- Does he or she address your whole health and not just your HIV status?

YOUR FIRST DOCTOR VISIT

Your first visit to the HIV specialist you've selected to oversee your care is a very important one. First, you'll be establishing a new relationship with someone with whom you'll be working to make informed decisions about your treatment for a very long time, perhaps for the rest of your life. It's likely that you'll be very anxious, and the doctor probably will anticipate this and try to reassure you, that despite your diagnosis, you can lead a healthy and productive life. This is a good time for you to ask questions, so you may want to jot down whatever questions you may have and take them with you to the appointment.

In addition to asking you questions about your medical history, the doctor will do a physical examination and order a number of blood tests. These blood tests will help your doctor to determine how the virus is affecting your body and whether you'll need to start treatment soon. The two standard tests include a CD4 count and a viral load test. The CD4 count reports the number of CD4 cells (or T cells) in a sample of your blood. The higher the count, the better the result, as CD4 cells are the white blood cells that fight infection, but are targeted by the HIV virus. The viral load test measures the amount of HIV in a sample of your blood. It shows how well your immune system is controlling the virus. The lower the load, the better the result. Together, the CD4 count and the viral load count provide a baseline (or initial) measurement for future tests.[11]

---

11 "HIV and Its Treatment: What You Should Know. Health Information for Patients," July2006. Published by the U.S. Department of Health and Human Services.

Your doctor is also likely to order drug resistance tests, which determine whether someone's HIV has developed resistance to any anti-HIV medication.[12] You may wonder how your virus could be resistant to anti-HIV medications before you've even taken them. The answer is that drug resistance is transmitted along with the virus. In other words, you will inherit whatever drug resistance the person who infected you with HIV has. Your doctor may also do other tests, including:

- A complete blood count (CBC), which checks all the different types of blood cells.

- A blood chemistry profile, which shows how well your liver and kidney are working, and measures the lipids (fats) and sugar (glucose) in your blood.

- Tests for other sexually transmitted diseases (STDs)

- Tests for other infections, like hepatitis, tuberculosis, or toxoplasmosis.[13]

If you're female, your doctor is also likely to order a pregnancy test and a Pap smear.

---

12 Ibid

13 Ibid.

BEGINNING TREATMENT

Depending on the results of these blood tests, you and your doctor will determine when you should start treatment and what medication to take. Not everyone who tests positive for HIV begins treatment right away. However, left untreated, HIV progresses into AIDS in an average of ten years. This rate of progression is a general estimate. HIV affects everyone differently. For a few people, referred to as the elite, HIV never progresses to AIDS. The National Institutes of Health recommends beginning treatment if:

- You are experiencing severe symptoms of HIV or have been diagnosed with AIDS.
- Your viral load is 100,000 copies/mL or more.
- Your CD4 count is 200 cells/mm^3 or less.[14]

Of course, you and your doctor may decide to begin taking the medication before any of these criteria are met.

MEDICINES THAT HELP

Anti-HIV medications are also known as antiretroviral medications. These are used to control the reproduc-

---

14 Ibid.

tion of the virus, thereby slowing the progression of HIV-related disease. To date, the U.S. Food and Drug Administration (FDA) has approved twenty-two antiretrovirals, which fall into four categories based on how they work against HIV. The four categories of antiretrovirals are:

- Nonnucleoside Reverse Transcriptase Inhibitors (NNRTIs)

- Nucleoside Reverse Transcriptase Inhibitors (NRTIs)

- Protease Inhibitors (PIs)

- Fusion Inhibitors

Nonnucleoside Reverse Transcriptase Inhibitors (NNRTIs) interrupt the first step HIV takes to copy itself, by binding to and disabling reverse transcriptase, a protein necessary to the copying process. NNRTIs include:

- Rescriptor (delavirdine)

- Viramune (nevirapine)

- Sustiva (efavirenz)

According to the FDA, Nucleoside Reverse Transcriptase Inhibitors (NRTIs) "are faulty versions of building blocks that HIV needs to make more copies of itself. When HIV uses an NRTI instead of a normal building block, reproduction of the virus is stalled." Like the NNRTIs, NRTIs also interrupt the first step HIV takes to copy itself. They include:

- AZT (zidovudine)
- Videx (didanosine)
- Ziagen (abacavir)
- Epivir (lamivudine)
- Emtriva (emtricitabine)
- Zerit (stavudine)
- Viread (tenofovir DF)
- Hivid (zalcitabine)
- Epzicom (a combination of Ziagen and Epivir)
- Combivir (a combination of Epivir and AZT)

- Trizivir (a combination of Ziagen, Epivir, and AZT)

- Truvada (a combination of Emtriva and Viread)

Protease Inhibitors (PIs) interrupt the last stage HIV takes to copy itself by disabling protease, a protein necessary for the copying process. It includes:

- Agenerase (amprenavir)

- Reyataz (atazanavir)

- Prezista (darunavir)

- Lexiva (fosamprenavir)

- Crixivan (indinavir)

- Viracept (nelfinavir)

- Norvir (ritonavir)

- Invirase (saquinavir)

- Aptivus (tipranavir)

- Kaletra (a combination of Norvir and a drug called Lopinavir)

Fusion Inhibitors work by blocking HIV from entering into cells. The FDA, to date, has approved only one drug in this class: Fuzeon (enfuvirtide).[15]

A Note About AZT

On March 20, 1987, AZT (zidovudine) became the first drug that the FDA approved to treat HIV/AIDS. Until the arrival of other antiretrovirals, it was administered in much higher dosages than it is today, typically one 400mg dose every four hours, even at night.* This rigid regimen, combined with the drug's toxic side effects, made it difficult for HIV patients to follow. Nevertheless, its effectiveness in slowing down the rate at which HIV reproduces itself lengthened the lives of HIV patients, bringing hope to patients and doctors alike. AZT also decreases the number of opportunistic infections, which means the person with HIV is less likely to have a number of illnesses at once. Another effect of AZT is to protect the brain against damage from the virus. As well, AZT is effective for reducing by two-thirds the risk of transmission of HIV from a pregnant woman to her baby; infection is less likely, but still happens about 25 percent of the time.

[* "Zidovudine." Wikipedia.com. Retrieved August 2006 (http://en.wikipedia.org/wiki/Zidovudine).]

---

15 Ibid.

Over time, doctors realized that HIV could gain an increased resistance to AZT over prolonged use. HIV makes small changes, or mutations, to its RNA. These mutations mean there may be several slightly different versions of HIV in one person's body, some resistant to one antibody or one drug. One drug alone may not be enough to stop the reproduction of all the versions of HIV. Fortunately, the development of other antiretrovirals allows AZT to be effective in combination with other drugs at smaller doses.

HAART

Today, the U.S. Department of Health and Human Services recommends a combination (or cocktail) of three or more medications in a regimen called Highly Active Antiretroviral Therapy (HAART). The wide number of antiretrovirals available allows your doctor and you to tailor your combination depending on your unique needs. Some of the factors to consider when choosing your combination are:

- The number of pills
- How often the pills must be taken
- Whether or not the pill should be taken with food
- How the medications interact with one another and with other medications you take

- The result of your drug resistance testing
- Other diseases and conditions you may have
- Pregnancy
- The combination's long-term effect on your body[16]

HAART regimens can reduce the level of HIV in your blood by more than 99 percent, thereby making your viral load undetectable, or too low to measure. When this happens, it becomes much harder for the virus to mutate, and if the virus cannot mutate, it cannot become resistant to the drugs.[17] This is why it is so important for you to take your medications as prescribed. Missing just a few doses a month can allow HIV to become resistant to the drugs. Also, pay attention to food requirements: your medication may not work as well if you ignore requirements to take it with food. If you experience side effects that you cannot tolerate, speak to your doctor about changing your regimen. Here are a few tips that you may use to help you to remember to take your dose on time.

---

16 "HIV and Its Treatment: What You Should Know. Health Information for Patients."

17 New York State Department of Health. "Staying on Schedule: Taking Your HIV Medicines."

- Make dose packs of the pills you need to take each day.
- Carry an extra dose with you in case you can't get home in time.
- Set your watch, phone, and/or iPod alarm for the times you need to take your medication.
- Associate taking your pill with a daily activity such as eating your dinner, brushing your teeth, or leaving for work.
- Have a friend call you to remind you to take your pill.
- Refill your prescription a week before you run out.

If you miss a dose, take it as soon as you remember, unless it is close to the time to take your next dose. Do not double your dose. Keep track of the doses you miss so that you can see how well you're doing. If you find that you're missing too many doses, it may be time to discuss changing your regimen with your doctor.

OTHER MEDICINES

Depending on your other health concerns, your doctor may prescribe medication that is not directly related to your HIV status. For example, antibiotics can be helpful, also, to cure diseases that strike when a person's immune system is not working well. Opportunistic infections take advantage of the opportunity of no resistance and are no longer small health problems. Some of these opportunistic infections are merely uncomfortable, like thrush, an infection of *Candida* yeast in the mouth. Others can be fatal if untreated. Often it is an opportunistic infection that kills a person with AIDS. Even vitamin pills can help a person with HIV to remain as well as possible for as long as possible. Vitamins and antibiotics are surprisingly helpful treatments for people who did not have good health before becoming infected with HIV.

FOLLOW-UP VISITS

Especially after you begin taking antiretroviral medications, you will be required to visit your doctor every three or four months so that he or she can monitor how well your treatment is working. During these visits, your doctor will order a CD4 count and a viral load test to measure against the baseline measurements that were established during your first visit. As well, he or she will monitor your general health.

You should use these scheduled visits to further develop your relationship with your doctor. When he or she asks you how things are going, be prepared to give him or her a full account of your health over the last few months. Consider making a list of the questions and issues you want to raise with your doctor. It may help you to keep a diary, noting the following:

- Missed doses
- New or changed symptoms that you've experienced since your last visit
- Major changes in your life that may affect your level of stress
- Your lab results (CD4, viral load, etc.)
- Other medications, vitamins, nutritional supplements that you're taking

TEN QUESTIONS TO ASK YOUR DOCTOR ABOUT HIV

1. What are the risks and benefits of HIV treatment?
2. What other diseases am I at risk for?
3. How can I avoid transmitting HIV to others?

4. How can I achieve and maintain a healthier lifestyle?

5. What should I do if I miss a dose of my HIV medication?

6. What should I do if I have problems sticking to my treatment regimen?

7. Can I infect someone else if my viral load is undetectable?

8. What are the likely side effects of the medications I take? Which side effects are serious?

9. Will the side effects go away by themselves? Are there any side effects that should prompt me to stop taking my medication?

10. How do I know if the drugs aren't working anymore?

CHAPTER SIX

Living with HIV/AIDS

JUST KNOWING THAT OTHER PEOPLE ARE FACING THE SAME CHALLENGES CAN HELP YOU FEEL LESS ISOLATED OR LONELY.

Finding out that you're HIV positive will definitely change your life. Especially after you begin treatment, HIV likely will factor into your everyday schedule in many ways. But your HIV status need not dominate your life, and the sooner you get used to your new routine, the better you'll be able to enjoy the rest of your life. There are many things you can do to maintain or improve your quality of life. Perhaps the most important ones are making sure that you stay healthy, developing a good support system, pursuing your dreams, and making time for fun.

GOOD HEALTH IS GOOD IN GENERAL

Of course, it is crucial that you follow your doctor's advice and keep your medical appointments. If you are taking prescription drugs, you must be careful to take every dose, as missed doses make the drugs less effective. However, there's more to being healthy than simply taking your "meds."

Diet and Exercise

Eating well and exercising are good for everyone in general, regardless of HIV status. However, they are even more essential for HIV-positive individuals, whose immune systems are constantly under assault by the virus. Becoming familiar with the U.S. Department of Agriculture's Food Guide Pyramid is a good place to start on your way to eating healthy. The pyramid shows that a balanced diet is one that includes all the major food groups but emphasizes certain foods (fruits, vegetables, grains, and dairy foods) over others (meat and oils). The pyramid also recommends at least thirty minutes of moderate to vigorous physical activity every day. Examples of moderate exercise include walking briskly, dancing, and bicycling. Vigorous exercise includes running, swimming, and basketball.*

[* U.S. Department of Agriculture, "Inside the Pyramid." Mypyramid.gov. Retrieved August 2006 (http://www.mypyramid.gov/pyramid/index.html)]

According to nutritionist Alan Lee, new studies show that the use of vitamin and mineral supplements offers benefits to people living with HIV. He says, "By getting enough vitamins and minerals through food and supplements, you will be helping your immune system and your overall health." His list of foods loaded with vitamins and minerals include butternut squash, yams, watermelon, fish, whole-grain cereal, sweet potatoes, peaches, oatmeal, 1 percent milk, collard greens, whole-wheat pasta, kale, pumpkin, oranges, wild rice, and chicken. He offers a guide to buying and using basic vitamin and mineral supplements:

- Look for a complete list of nutrients on the label that supply 100 percent of the "Daily Value."
- Look for "USP" on the label to make sure you're getting what the label actually states.
- Always take your vitamins with food.
- Take your vitamins with your HIV medications, unless your medications require that you take them on an empty stomach.
- Discuss your vitamin and mineral supplementation plan with your doctor to make sure that your supplements don't interact with your medications.[18]

When the kitchen door slammed, Tyler shouted up the basement stairs to the kitchen. "Holly? Are you home from school?"

Holly put down her knapsack. "Yeah. What is it?"

---

18 Alan Lee, "Update on Vitamins & Minerals: What and How Much to Take." HIV Positive!, June/July 2006, pp.28–31.

"Can you help me carry my hockey gear upstairs?" he asked.

"Sure." Holly came downstairs and took one handle of the big duffle bag. Carrying it between them, they got the bag of gear upstairs.

"Sorry I can't do this by myself," said Tyler. "I don't want to bother you."

"I don't mind," Holly told him. "When I was a little baby, you used to carry me everywhere. Are you playing hockey tonight? You haven't been to a game for a while."

"No, I'm not planning to play it anymore," said Tyler. "I'm selling my gear for cheap to a guy who is joining the team."

"But you love playing hockey with your friends!" Holly protested. "Did somebody say something to make you quit?"

Tyler laughed. "No, they've been great since last year when I told them I'm HIV positive. But the last couple of times I played, I got some bruises that took a long time to get better. I don't hurt like that after riding my bike. I'm going riding on Saturdays with two of the guys.

They say cross-training will make them stronger for hockey."

"If bike riding makes you stronger, too, then that's good," said Holly. "Maybe if we fix the flat tire on my old bike, you and I can go for a ride sometime."

Avoiding Risky Behaviors

Of course, good general health includes avoiding risky behavior. Being HIV positive doesn't give you a free pass to continue or start sharing needles during drug use or having unprotected sex. On the contrary, having HIV is a strong reason not to engage in these behaviors. In addition to exposing others to infection, you run the risk of superinfection, which is becoming infected with another strain of HIV. Superinfection increases the likelihood of your developing resistance to anti-HIV medication, which will reduce the treatment options available to you.

Moreover, drug abuse, whether or not it involves needles, impairs a person's good judgment. A person who abuses drugs may end up doing other dangerous things as well. There is the risk of addiction and immediate death. In addition, a person who abuses drugs is at greater risk of being beaten or raped, of catching many kinds of diseases, or of being injured. These are avoidable risks.

A person's immune system may be weakened by drug abuse. This can make it easier to become ill with many kinds of diseases, including AIDS. Drug abuse can also interfere with the medicines prescribed by a doctor. It's important to be honest with your doctor about any substance use, whether it's a lot or a little, and whether it's alcohol, illegal drugs, misused prescription drugs, or marijuana. Even cigarettes and tobacco, though legal, are addictive and have profound health effects. If you are abusing intravenous drugs or any substance, consider seeking help.

IDENTIFY YOURSELF

People living with HIV should consider wearing a MedicAlert tag. It can be worn as a bracelet or necklace. Many people wear them for many health reasons. In case of an accident, emergency workers always look to see if a person is wearing a MedicAlert tag. Any doctor's office or clinic, and even most drugstores, will have information on how to register for a MedicAlert tag.

A MedicAlert tag can be something you show to one person in a crowded room, for example, if you need to tell a nurse you are HIV positive, but don't feel like saying it out loud for everyone in the waiting room to hear.

If someone peeks at your MedicAlert tag and asks why you are wearing it, you have a choice. You can tell them the reason, let them read it, or quietly say that it's private.

HOW TO PROTECT OTHERS

If you are HIV positive, you have a responsibility not to infect other people with the virus. Be honest about your HIV status. People who care about you deserve to know this. It's hard to risk rejection, but being honest is being responsible.

- Tell your sexual partner that you are HIV positive.
- Do not have unprotected sex, even if you previously had unprotected sex with this person.
- Tell people with whom you have had sex that you are HIV positive.
- If you hope to have a new sexual partner, tell this person you are HIV positive before becoming intimate.
- Do not share your razor or toothbrush with anyone.

- If you become pregnant, or if you are thinking about having a child, talk to your doctor right away.

- If you abuse drugs, do not share needles. More important, get help for your addiction.

GETTING SUPPORT

Did you ever help a member of your family who was sick? Or did you lift some heavy things for someone older or pregnant? Maybe you were the person who taught your younger relatives how to ride a bicycle. If you have ever done anything like this, or had someone help you, you know that when one person needs help, it can affect many people who care.

Everybody needs help of some kind sooner or later, even big, strong people who can work hard and never seem to get sick with even a cold. Some kinds of physical help are obvious, but emotional help and encouragement is real, too. We get most of the help we need from our friends and family because that's one of the things we do when we care about each other.

Some people are ashamed to ask for help or to need help at all. We have to try not to embarrass each other and simply do what is needed without making any fuss about it. You were born a tiny baby who needed help, and you can hope to live a long time before needing that much help again. In the meantime, you can help others.

Emotional and Spiritual Support

When people need health care, they also need emotional and spiritual care. There are many kinds of support available. Having emotional and spiritual support can not only make you feel better in your mind, it can help your physical health as well.

Some people get the support they need from religious faith, others from psychology and scientific disciplines. You may want to consider traditional supports already in use by your family and culture. Perhaps you will find alternative methods more helpful. There are libraries and resource centers to consult, and you may get good recommendations from your friends and health care providers.

If you have a good emotional and spiritual adviser, that person will work to help you live well, even though HIV/AIDS is affecting your life, your family, and your community.

Support Groups

There are support groups for people living with AIDS and HIV. Support groups can bring you a great deal of comfort as you meet people who share similar emotions and experiences. Just knowing that other people are facing the same challenges can help you feel less isolated or lonely.

The people in a support group are people like yourself, whose lives are affected by HIV and AIDS. They can help you understand treatment methods and ways to adjust your lifestyle. Usually one of them will have some training as a facilitator and will be able to help find resources or the answers to questions. Some people prefer to ask questions or express their worries in a support group, rather than at home.

It can make you feel isolated and alone if you are HIV positive and have not told your family. If you're scared of what they will say, or you are just not yet ready to share, that's understandable. A support group can help you prepare yourself for how you will tell your friends and family.

You can be affected by AIDS, even if you are not the person infected with HIV. Finding out that someone you care about is HIV positive is very upsetting. Support groups help friends and family as well, not only the person who is HIV positive.

Physical Care

A person who is HIV positive but at an asymptomatic stage may not need much physical help at all. However, for someone who is at an early symptomatic stage, there may be times when he or she needs assistance for daily living. On occasion, the care of a trained nurse may be needed, but friends or family can often learn how to care for the majority of a person's physical needs.

By the time a person is diagnosed with AIDS, there will be good days and bad days, but the person is likely to need physical care much of the time. Family members and friends can take turns helping where needed. Or perhaps one helper will concentrate on one aspect, like running errands and doing laundry, while another will look after nursing care.

The changes in what a person is physically able to do can be very upsetting for everyone. It can also be an opportunity to recognize that we all live in real bodies, bodies that change with time and health and chance. There will certainly be emotional reactions as well.

Emotional Effects

It is emotionally exhausting when anyone in a household is ill. And when illnesses go on for months or years, the entire household must make adjustments and plan ways to renew each person's emotional strength. Take time to restore your own energy, and make sure everyone in your household does the same. This is one way you can help each other. You can also give each other space to feel better.

Support groups can be a great help. A support group may suggest ideas that worked in other households. The members may offer validation that your emotional reactions are realistic, not whining or selfish or unreasonable. Sometimes part of the solution is just knowing that other people are going through similar experiences.

When a Hospice Is the Answer

People living with AIDS often rely on hospice organizations. A hospice can be a palliative care hospital, where people go for nursing care when they are dying. The hospice organization can also be for people who want to be in control of their lives as they confront their terminal illnesses.

In a hospice program, the doctors, registered nurses, counselors, and social workers work with a patient and his or her own doctor to manage pain and plan treatments. They provide advice and support. Most of their services are offered at the patient's home.

There are more than 3,000 hospice programs in the United States, providing care for at least half a million people.

What Difference Can I Make?

You are only one person. But each day, you can do something positive to make that day better. Even small improvements are real and can be special.

You may be able to work together with a circle of family and friends to accomplish things that make your lives better. You may be part of a larger project or political movement that influences the lives of many people. Anything that changes the world happens because of the actions of individual people.

You have the ability to be nice to the people who live in your home. A kind word, helping someone with homework or housework, telling a funny story, or listening to someone else's news: these are all things that show that you care. They can be done even by a person who usually needs the most help from the others.

DISCLOSING YOUR HIV STATUS

Being HIV positive isn't something that will be obvious to everyone. Even having AIDS is not as visible as losing an arm or using a wheelchair. It is a health difference that doesn't show, and it's up to you to decide what difference it makes in the ways you behave with the people you meet.

It's not your job to educate everybody you see about AIDS and HIV. But it doesn't hurt to think ahead once in a while. What would you say if someone asked you a question? How could you help a stranger who had an accident? When is it best to be anonymous?

Some days you will make different decisions about what to say and what actions to take. But you can always use your knowledge about HIV and AIDS to help you be confident that you are making good decisions for your health and for your community.

Does Everyone Know?

If you live in a large city, probably no one at all will know if you are HIV positive, unless you have told them yourself. Don't be self-conscious about how you look, or whether anyone can tell. Don't waste a lot of time wondering if strangers are looking at you or thinking about you. Just go about your activities as you normally do. Nobody can tell just from looking at you.

If you live in a small town or very connected neighborhood, everyone you meet casually might know if you are HIV positive because you and your family may have told them. If you don't know how you feel about that, remember that you probably know something about many of them as well. Many people will try to be polite or nice. However, some won't.

Some people who are HIV positive or have AIDS find it easier to share the news with a group (perhaps at church, school, or a community center), rather than to try to keep it a secret. This sharing can be a way to be confident in the company of your neighbors. It can also be a way to learn who is afraid of the disease or ignorant. Perhaps your group will ask a health center to hold an information session for the community. However, you should always be aware that by disclosing your status, you risk rejection.

PROTECTION FROM DISCRIMINATION

There are laws in the United States and Canada that make it illegal to discriminate against anyone on the basis of race, creed, color, and sex; these laws also ensure that people with HIV or AIDS are protected from discrimination. In 1990, the U.S. Congress passed the Americans with Disabilities Act. This act specifically prohibits discrimination against anyone with HIV or AIDS.*

[* U.S. Department of Justice, "Questions and Answers: The Americans with Disabilities Act and Persons with HIV/AIDS." Retrieved August 2006 (http://www.usdoj.gov/crt/ada/pubs/hivqanda.txt).]

That is the law. But in practice, there are still many ignorant people who are prejudiced against things they don't understand. AIDS is scary enough without people treating each other badly.

You will probably see prejudice and discrimination happening. Sometimes you will be able to improve a situation right away. Sometimes your efforts will have more results if you work as part of a group, for education or justice or one small improvement. It is not your responsibility to solve everybody else's prejudice.

BEING AN EXAMPLE

Some things about AIDS and HIV are private. But there are also times when it is proper to speak in public about AIDS, go to a meeting, or march in a parade. A loop of red ribbon pinned on a shirt or jacket is a visible reminder that you care.

There are activities you can do with other people in your community to show support for people with HIV or AIDS. There are educational programs. Some communities have fund-raising events to raise money for a local clinic or hospice. Other programs send money overseas to support people with AIDS/HIV or their orphaned children. There is an art exhibit of quilts designed to commemorate people with AIDS, called the AIDS Memorial Quilt, which tours North America.

The late Princess Diana was the first wife of Charles, the Prince of Wales. Photographers used to follow her almost everywhere because her husband was the heir to the British throne, and also because she became an icon in her own right. When visiting hospitals, Princess Diana would shake hands with people who had AIDS. Though photographers made her uncomfortable, she made sure that pictures were taken of these handshakes. Because her photographs appeared in many newspapers, she hoped this would help people understand that we don't have to be afraid to talk to and touch someone who has AIDS.

MYTHS AND FACTS ABOUT HIV/AIDS

Myth: AIDS is only a problem for gay people.

Fact: HIV/AIDS is something for everyone to know about, whether they are homosexual or heterosexual. Even people who never have sex may someday need a blood transfusion, and they will be glad to receive blood that has been tested for HIV antibodies.

Myth: AIDS is only a problem in crowded cities.

Fact: AIDS is a problem wherever people are. People can be exposed to HIV one time and after that can take the virus wherever they go.

Myth: Kids don't have to worry about AIDS.

Fact: Babies can be born HIV positive. Children can be infected with HIV just like adults can.

Myth: AIDS is a special punishment for doing wrong.

Fact: AIDS is a disease and not a punishment.

Myth: All the people who get AIDS have done such bad things that they all deserve to get sick and die.

Fact: Nobody gets sick from anything just because he or she deserves it. Some people who do bad things get sick. Some people who get sick never did any bad things at all. Some people who do bad things never get sick. If people only ever got sick and died when they deserved it, we would all know.

Myth: Nobody cares about those people who have AIDS.

Fact: There are programs to help people with HIV or AIDS all over North America, through the United Nations, and around the world. Some programs concentrate on prevention and education. Others work with people who are already ill and with their families. These programs are staffed with volunteers and health care professionals who care.

Myth: Even if I abuse drugs, I can't get AIDS unless I share a needle with another user.

Fact: Drug abusers can become infected with HIV by sharing needles or doing other high-risk activities while they are under the influence of the drugs. Drug abusers can have plenty of diseases and health problems, even if they don't share needles. They are also at risk for dangerous behavior and violent crimes.

Myth: If kids learn anything about sex, they are more likely to have sex and get AIDS.

Fact: Sexual health education helps young people understand their bodies and how to stay healthy.

Myth: Maybe a sick person with AIDS could get cured by having sex with a virgin.

Fact: Nothing cures AIDS. If a person with any disease has sex with a virgin, that does not cure any disease. It may even give the disease to the virgin.

Myth: My friend is so clean and smart. He would never have AIDS.

Fact: You can't tell if a person is HIV positive just by how he looks or talks or thinks. You have to ask. And anyone who has done any high-risk behavior should have an HIV test.

Myth: Once people get AIDS, they are going to die soon. Nothing can be done.

Fact: Some people who have HIV can live for years with good medical care and good nutrition. They can even enjoy moderately good health and most normal activities. Some have lived fifteen years or more without progressing to a diagnosis of AIDS.

CHAPTER SEVEN

HIV/AIDS Around the World

HALF OF ALL PEOPLE INFECTED BY THE VIRUS THAT CAUSES AIDS ARE AGED 15 TO 24 YEARS.

AIDS is a problem facing every nation in the world. The governments of many countries have responded to the AIDS crisis by making careful plans intended to protect their citizens' health. Education and prevention are two of the major efforts. Medical treatment is usually made available for people who are HIV positive or who have AIDS. The United Nations (UN) and the World Health Organization (WHO) are working with nations on the issue.

As of 2005, an estimated 40.3 million people around the world are infected with HIV, and 90 percent of those people live in developing countries, according to UNAIDS, an alliance of six United Nations agencies. It is further estimated that 3 million people will die of AIDS in 2006.*

[* UNAIDS/WHO AIDS Epidemic Update: December 2005 (http://www.unaids.org/epi/2005/doc/EPIupdate2005_html_en/epi05_03_en.htm).]

STATISTICS BY REGION

Unfortunately, as these statistics reveal, the countries that are most affected by HIV/AIDS often lack the resources to provide proper care for their citizens. Moreover, efforts by international health agencies and charitable organizations often come up against entrenched social and cultural obstacles as they try to alleviate the suffering of HIV/AIDS patients in developing nations. Nevertheless, these organizations continue in their quest to raise public awareness about AIDS and how it can be prevented, to reduce the fear and stigma surrounding the disease, and to bring treatment and comfort to HIV/AIDS patients in even the most remote regions.

Their reports are simultaneously encouraging and heartbreaking: News of success in raising awareness, changing attitudes, and saving lives in a region falls within the context of the terrible toll of the disease on its population. So, these organizations continue to urge developed nations to offer more funds to combat the disease. They also continue to encourage large pharmaceutical companies to provide expensive anti-HIV drugs to poor countries at significantly reduced costs.

Of the more than 40 million people estimated by the UN to be living with HIV in 2005, the numbers living in various regions are as follows:

Region	Living with HIV	Newly Infected
North America	1.2 million	43,000
Caribbean	300,000	30,000
Latin America	1.8 million	200,000
Western and Central Europe	720,000	22,000
North Africa and the Mideast	510,000	67,000
Sub-Saharan Africa	25.8 million	3.2 million
Eastern Europe and Central Asia	1.6 million	207,000
South and Southeast Asia	7.4 million	990,000
East Asia	870,000	140,000
Australia and Oceania	74,000	8,200

UNDERSTANDING THE DISTRIBUTION

Though AIDS began as a rare infection in West Africa some fifty years ago, there are now people dying of AIDS in every part of the world. No region is free of the virus that causes AIDS. But the risk of AIDS is not distributed evenly around the world, just as the resources to prevent or treat AIDS are not evenly distributed. When we look at the statistics for who is becoming infected with HIV, we can see that the rate varies from region to region.

The variation is not just due to population density. There are densely populated places that have lower rates of HIV infection per 1,000 residents. These places are usually in industrialized nations.

The variation also isn't due to some places being isolated, with few visitors. Just a few visitors are enough to bring HIV into an isolated region. The variation is largely due to how many people have been educated about how HIV is transmitted.

When people are taught that AIDS is caused by HIV and how the virus can pass from person to person, the rate of new HIV infections drops in that area. When these people also have access to condoms and are encouraged by their families and local authorities not to have unprotected sex outside of marriage, the rate of new HIV infections drops further, close to the rate seen in industrialized nations.

LIFE EXPECTANCY IS AFFECTED BY AIDS

Africa, with only about 10 percent of the world's population, suffers more than half of the world's total HIV infections. In many African countries south of the Sahara desert, the average life expectancy is dropping because so many people are dying of AIDS. The World Health Organization announced in its 2006 annual report that the average woman in Zimbabwe is dying at age thirty-four. Men in Zimbabwe can expect to live only to age thirty-seven, on average.

There has been some progress made in Kenya and Uganda in reducing the numbers of people newly infected with HIV each year. But in South Africa, 20 percent of the population between the ages of fifteen and forty-nine is carrying HIV. This is an increase from only 1 percent in 1990.[19]

Health care services in many African countries are overwhelmed and are simply unable to handle all the people who need basic care. Few people in developing countries are able to afford treatment to keep a person who is HIV positive from progressing to full-blown AIDS. Sometimes antibiotics and even vitamins are simply not available or affordable.

THE OBSTACLE IS COST

The obstacle to treating AIDS with any medication is cost. A year's worth of daily AZT doses can cost up to $6,000. Triple-drug therapy can cost $16,000 a year.[20] In North America, many private insurance companies and government-funded medical insurance programs cover some AIDS treatments.

---

19 Ibid.

20 White, Katherine. Everything You Need to Know About AIDS and HIV. New York, NY: The Rosen Publishing Group, 2001.

The cost of treatment is even more of a problem in developing countries. The drugs cannot be afforded by any but the wealthiest people, and their governments cannot afford to provide treatment either.

PREVENTION IS A WORTHY EXPENSE

A health care nurse may not charge anyone for a lesson in how to prevent HIV infection, but a community can find it hard to support the nurse's wages. Even the cost of condoms is more than many people in developing countries can afford. There are programs being developed by the United Nations and volunteer agencies to make condoms affordable or free and easily available. Although 95 percent of people living with AIDS reside in developing countries, 95 percent of AIDS prevention money is spent in industrial countries.*

[* Food and Agricultural Organization of the United Nations. "Three UN Agencies Join Hands in the Fight Against HIV/AIDS." FAO.org. Retrieved August 2006 (http://www.fao.org.waicent/OIS/PRESS_NE/PRESSENG/2001/pren0195.htm).]

The U.S. government made a pledge in 2003 to spend $15 billion for AIDS prevention in fifteen of the most heavily affected countries of the world. In

2006, $3.2 billion will be spent, up from $2.6 billion in 2005. At the core of these efforts is a program called A-B-C, which stresses abstinence, being faithful in marriage, and using condoms correctly.*

[* AIDS in America and AIDS in Canada Free Health Software. University of Alberta Health Info Site. Accessed March 6, 2006 (http://www.uofaweb.ualberta.ca/healthinfo/nav02.cfm?nav02=27904&nav01=27613).]

ORPHANED BY AIDS

In some developing countries, when parents have died of AIDS, their orphaned children are particularly vulnerable to this disease and other health problems because of poverty. When there is a grandparent or other relative who is able to help, often their family resources are stretched too far to be able to feed, shelter, and provide for everyone adequately. Children can end up alone or caring for their younger siblings.

There are efforts being made to help children orphaned by AIDS, whether or not they are HIV positive themselves. Orphanages and schools can make a big difference in these children's lives. Private agencies, volunteer groups, and faith-based organizations are working together to try to provide for these children's needs.

YOUNG PEOPLE ARE PARTICULARLY VULNERABLE

"Half of all people infected with the virus that causes AIDS are aged 15 to 24 years," says Susan Lee in her article "AIDS: Young People Dying of Embarrassment—HIV Report." She says these young people are "victims of their exclusion from prevention strategies and of cultural mores against discussing sexual matters."*

[* Susan Lee, "Aids: Young People Dying of Embarrassment—HIV Report." Common Dreams News Center. Retrieved January 2006 (http://www.commondreams.org).]

In many countries around the world, it is hard for people to talk about sex and sexually transmitted diseases. Some cultures believe that it is just not proper to talk about sexual matters at all. But what is wrong is for anyone to die from a disease that he or she could have learned to avoid.

UNITED NATIONS COMMITS TO EDUCATING YOUNG PEOPLE

The United Nations (UN) maintains the Interagency Task Team on HIV/AIDS and Young People. As well, conferences for health ministers are held regularly. The benefits of research, statistics, and methods by UN programs are made available internationally.

In June 2001, the United Nations held a special session on HIV/AIDS in New York. Delegates at the general assembly made the Declaration of Commitment on HIV/AIDS: Global Targets for Young People. They dedicated regional and worldwide efforts to preventing HIV transmission among young people. Their goal was:

> By 2005, ensure that at least 90 percent, and by 2010 at least 95 percent of young men and women aged 15 to 24 have access to information, education, including peer and youth-specific HIV education, and services necessary to develop the life skills required to reduce their vulnerability to HIV infection, in full partnership with young persons, parents, families, educators and healthcare providers.*

[* United Nations General Assembly Special Session on HIV/AIDS. "Declaration of Commitment on HIV/AIDS: Global Targets for Young People, Dedicating Regional and World-Wide Efforts to Preventing HIV Transmission Among Young People." New York, NY. June 2001. Retrieved August 2006 (http://www.unaids.org/en/Goals/UNGASS/default.asp).]

In Dublin, Ireland, in February 2004, the United Nations renewed that dedication at a ministerial conference called Breaking the Barriers—Partnership to Fight HIV/AIDS in Europe and Central Asia. Delegates resolved to "reinvigorate our efforts to ensure the target of the Declaration of Commitment."

AIDS IS A PROBLEM FOR EVERYONE

People who become infected with HIV may be rich or poor. But people who are wealthy can afford to make good health choices that make them less vulnerable to diseases in general, and HIV in particular. People who are poor can lack more than money to pay for education or buy condoms or medicine; they also can lack the ability and/or knowledge to protect their health from AIDS and other dangers.

When people have no education about AIDS/HIV, or have no ability to make good health choices, they are more likely to catch this or other diseases. Awareness programs must no longer be undermined by stigmas attached to AIDS. The more people who have education about AIDS/HIV, the fewer who will get the disease.

TEN FACTS ABOUT AIDS

1. More than 40 million people worldwide are living with HIV or AIDS.

2. You can't get AIDS from an insect bite.

3. Just one sexual contact or shared needle is enough to transmit HIV from person to person.

4. Having sex with a virgin will not cure AIDS or any other disease.

5. You don't have to be afraid to talk with and hold the hand of someone with AIDS.

6. Working with or living with someone who has AIDS will not spread the disease.

7. AIDS is a problem everywhere, not just in big cities or developing nations.

8. Doctors, nurses, and technicians are doing their part to keep medical procedures safe from risk of HIV infection.

9. Tests for HIV are available around the world; you can be tested easily.

10. An HIV-positive individual who gets good medical care can live for many years before developing AIDS.

GLOSSARY

abstinence Refraining from sexual intercourse.

AIDS Acquired immunodeficiency syndrome; a disease caused by HIV. It is usually diagnosed when a person's T-helper cell count drops below 200.

anonymous HIV testing A type of HIV testing in which the person tested is assigned a unique code that is used for identification instead of his or her name; the test results are completely confidential.

antibiotics Drugs used to treat infection.

antibody A substance made by a person's T-cells to fight a particular infection.

asymptomatic The presence of an illness without any symptoms.

bacteria Microscopic single-cell organisms, some of which can cause diseases.

blood transfusion The transfer of blood or blood products from one person to another.

CD4 count A test done to count the number of T-cells in the immune system of a person with HIV or AIDS.

chemotherapy The treatment of cancer using drugs that are intended to destroy malignant cells.

confidential HIV testing A type of HIV test that uses the name of the person tested and releases the name and results to the person's doctor; also called names testing.

contagious Able to be passed from one person to another.

dementia A significant decline in mental abilities, including memory loss and the ability to take care of one's self.

dental dam A square piece of latex usually used in dental procedures, but which can be used to practice safe sex.

diagnosis The identification of an illness.

DNA (deoxyribonucleic acid) The molecule inside the nucleus of a cell that carries the genetic instructions for making living organisms.

enzyme A protein that triggers chemical reactions in the body.

epidemic A widespread outbreak of an infectious disease.

extinct No longer existing.

fidelity An exclusive commitment to one romantic or sexual partner.

GRID Gay-related immune deficiency; an early term used for the disease now called AIDS.

hemophilia A genetic condition from birth in which a person's blood does not clot properly, causing excessive bleeding from a slight injury.

HIV Human immunodeficiency virus; the virus that causes AIDS.

immune system The body's defense system against illness, disease, and infection.

immunization Using a vaccine to stimulate the immune system to fight infection.

intravenous drug use Directly injecting drugs into the bloodstream by using a needle.

Kaposi's sarcoma A rare type of cancer causing skin lesions.

lubricant An oily or slippery substance used to reduce friction and trauma during sexual intercourse.

lymph node A small gland that makes up part of the body's immune system that fights against invading bacteria and foreign particles.

lymphoma A cancer of the lymphatic system.

mutate To change, as in the genetic material of a cell.

opportunistic infection An infection that occurs when organisms take advantage of a weakened immune system.

PCP (Pneumocystis carinii pneumonia) A form of pneumonia seen primarily in patients with weakened immune systems.

protease inhibitors A class of drugs that works to kill HIV when the virus is making copies of itself.

retrovirus A type of virus that has RNA instead of DNA as its genetic material.

RNA (ribonucleic acid) A chemical found in the nucleus and cytoplasm of cells that is similar to DNA. RNA is responsible for translating thegenetic code of DNA into proteins.

safe sex Sex that does not permit infections and illnesses to pass from one person to another; most often, sex that includes use of a condom or dental dam.

seroconversion The body's development of antibodies to fight against an invading microorganism.

spermicide A substance that kills sperm.

T-cell The type of white blood cell that produces antibodies.

T-helper cell A type of white blood cell that helps fight off bacteria and viruses that enter the body; the cell type that HIV attacks and destroys.

vertical transmission A term used to describe how HIV is passed from mother to unborn child.

virus A tiny germ that needs to enter the cells of a living organism to become activated and multiply.

white blood cells Cells that circulate in the bloodstream and lymph system throughout the body; part of the immune system that attacks foreign invaders of the body.

WHERE TO GO FOR HELP

AIDS Action Committee of Massachusetts, Inc.
294 Washington Street, 5th Floor
Boston, MA 02108
(617)437-6200
Web site: http://aac.org

The AIDS Action Committee of Massachusetts is New England's largest and oldest AIDS service organization.

AIDS Alliance for Children, Youth & Families
1600 K Street NW, Suite 200
Washington, DC 20006
(888)917-AIDS(2437)
Web site: http://www.aidsalliance.org

This nonprofit group focuses on the concerns of children, young adults, women, and families affected by HIV/AIDS.

AIDSinfo
P.O. Box 6303
Rockville, MD 20849-6303
(800)448-0440
Web site: http://www.aidsinfo.nih.gov

AIDSinfo is a U.S. Department of Health and Human Services project that offers information on HIV/AIDS treatment, prevention, and research.

American Social Health Association (ASHA)
P.O. Box 13827
Research Triangle Park, NC 27709
(919)361-8400
Web site: http://www.ashastd.org

The American Social Health Association is a nonprofit organization that provides information and service centers aimed at fighting the spread of sexually transmitted diseases.

The Black AIDS Institute
1833 West Eighth Street, #200
Los Angeles, CA 90057
(213)353-3610
Web site: http://www.blackaids.org

The Black Aids Institute seeks to reduce the disproportionately high incidence of HIV/AIDS among African Americans by mobilizing Black institutions and individuals to confront the disease in African American communities.

The Body
Body Health Resources Corporation
250 West 57th Street
New York, NY 10107
Web site: http://www.thebody.com/index.html

The Body offers comprehensive information on AIDS prevention, treatment, and research. Its Web site has a wealth of links to other AIDS organizations.

Canadian Aboriginal AIDS Network
602-251 Bank Street
Ottawa, ON K2P 1X3
Canada
(888)285-2226
Web site: http://www.caan.ca

A national coalition of Aboriginal people and organizations providing leadership, advocacy, and support for Aboriginal people living with and/or affected by HIV/AIDS.

Canadian AIDS Society
190 O'Connor Street, Suite 800
Ottawa, ON K2P 2R3
Canada
(800)499-1986,
Web site: http://www.cdnaids.ca

The Canadian AIDS Society is a network of more than 100 community-based AIDS organizations across Canada.

Canadian HIV/AIDS Information Centre
400-1565 Carling Avenue
Ottawa, ON K1Z 8R1

Canada
(877)999-7740
Web site: http://www.aidssida.cpha.ca

The Canadian HIV/AIDS Information Centre is the largest information center on HIV/AIDS in Canada.

Centers for Disease Control and Prevention (CDC)
1600 Clifton Road
Atlanta, GA 30333
(800)311-3435 (Public Inquiries)
(800)342-2437 (National AIDS hotline—English)
(800)344-7432 (National AIDS hotline—Spanish)
(800)243-7889 (National AIDS hotline—TTY)

The Centers for Disease Control and Prevention is the United States' main federal agency for protecting the health and safety of Americans. As such, it monitors and seeks to control the spread of diseases in the United States.

Gay Men's Health Crisis (GMHC)
The Tisch Building
119 West 24th Street
New York, NY 10011
(212)367-1000
Web site: http://www.gmhc.org

The Gay Men's Health Crisis was the first AIDS organization in the United States and the world. As such, it was at the forefront of the global fight against AIDS. It continues to raise awareness about the disease, particularly in gay and lesbian communities, and to fund AIDS research.

HIV *Positive!* Magazine
Positive Health Publications, Inc.
1374 Thornborough Drive
Alpharetta, GA 30004
(678)762-0821
Web site: http://hivpositivemagazine.com

Through both its print and online editions, *HIV Positive!* magazine publishes articles to help HIV/AIDS patients live healthy and productive lives.

National Native American AIDS Prevention Center (NNAAPC)
436 14th Street, Suite 1020
Oakland, CA 94612
(510)444-2051
Web site: http://www.nnaapc.org

Founded in 1987, the NNAAPC is a national nonprofit organization that works toward AIDS prevention and addresses the impact of HIV/AIDS on American Indians, native Alaskans, and native Hawaiians through culturally appropriate advocacy and research.

LIFEbeat, Inc.

630 9th Avenue, Suite 1010
New York, NY 10036
(212)459-2590
(800)AIDS-411(243-7411)
Web site: http://www.lifebeat.org

LIFEbeat's mission is to mobilize the talents and resources of the music industry to raise awareness about HIV/AIDS among American youth and to provide support to the AIDS community.

WEB SITES

Due to the changing nature of Internet links, Rosen Publishing has developed an online list of Web sites related to the subject of this book. This site is updated regularly. Please use this link to access the list:

http://www.rosenlinks.com/ccw/hiai

FOR FURTHER READING

Bardhan-Quallen, Sudipta. *AIDS.* Detroit, MI: KidHaven Press, 2005.

Cefrey, Holly. *AIDS. Epidemics: Deadly Diseases Throughout History.* New York, NY: Rosen Publishing, 2001.

Connolly, Sean. *AIDS.* Chicago, IL: Heinemann Library, 2003.

Critzer, Timothy. *HIV and Me: Firsthand Information for Coping with HIV and AIDS.* San Francisco, CA: Firsthand Books, 2004.

Derlega, Valerian J., and Anita P. Barbee, eds. *HIV and Social Interaction.* Thousand Oaks, CA: Sage Publications, 1998.

Grodeck, Brett, and Daniel S. Berger. *The First Year—HIV: An Essential Guide for the Newly Diagnosed.* New York, NY: Marlowe & Company, 2003.

Halpin, Mikki. *It's Your World—If You Don't Like It, Change It: Activism for Teenagers.* New York, NY: Simon Pulse, 2004.

Jenkins, Mark. *HIV/AIDS: Practical, Medical and Spiritual Guidelines for Daily Living When You're HIV-Positive.* Center City, MN: Hazelden, 2000.

Johnson, Earvin "Magic." *What You Can Do to Avoid AIDS.* New York, NY: New York Times Books, 1992.

Shein, Lori. *AIDS.* San Diego, CA: Lucent Books, Inc., 1998.

Taylor-Brown, Susan, and Alejandro Garcia, eds. *HIV Affected and Vulnerable Youth: Prevention Issues and Approaches.* New York, NY: Haworth Press, 1999.

Watstei, Sarah Barbara, and Stephen E. Stratton. *The Encyclopedia of HIV and AIDS.* New York, NY: Facts on File, 2003.

White, Katherine. *Everything You Need to Know About AIDS and HIV.* New York, NY: Rosen Publishing, 2001.

White, Ryan, and Marie Cunningham. *Ryan White, My Own Story.* New York, NY: Dial Books, 1991.

BIBLIOGRAPHY

AIDS in America and AIDS in Canada Free Health Software. University of Alberta Health Info Site. Accessed March 6, 2006 (http://www.uofaweb.ualberta.ca/healthinfo/nav02.cfm?nav02=27904&nav01=27613).

"AIDS Relentless March Leaves Legacy of Misery." Associated Press, June 5, 2006. Retrieved July 2006 (http://www.msnbc.msn.com/id/13072820).

The Body. "A Guide to HIV Drug Resistance." 2004.

Burns, Nick. "First Steps." *POZ,* November 2005, pp.4-5.

Burns, Nick. "Will I Still Have a Sex Life?" *POZ,* November 2005, pp.8-9.

Centers for Disease Control and Prevention. "Drug-Associated HIV Transmission Continues in the United States." May 2002. Retrieved August 2006 (http://www.cdc.gov/hiv/resources/factsheets/idu.htm).

Centers for Disease Control and Prevention. "HIV/AIDS Among Men Who Have Sex With Men." Retrieved July 2006 (http://www.cdc.gov/hiv/resources/factsheets/msm.htm).

Centers for Disease Control and Prevention. HIV/AIDS Surveillance Report 2004, Vol.16. Retrieved April 2006 (http://www.cdc.gov/hiv/topics/surveillance/resources/reports/2004report/default.htm).

Centers for Disease Control and Prevention. "Living with HIV/AIDS." Updated September 2005. Retrieved August 2006. (http://www.cdc.gov/hiv/pubs/brochure/livingwithhiv.htm).

DeNoon, Daniel. "CDC: Everyone to Get HIV Test." WebMD. Retrieved August 2006 (http://www.webmd.com/content/article/121/114438.htm).

Food and Agricultural Organization of the United Nations. "Three UN Agencies Join Hands in the Fight Against HIV/AIDS." FAO.org. Retrieved August 2006 (http://www.fao.org.waicent/OIS/PRESS_NE/PRESSENG/2001/pren0195.htm).

Highleyman, Liz. "Time for HIV Treatment." *POZ,* November 2005, pp.12–13.

"HIV and Its Treatment: What You Should Know. Health Information for Patients." July 2006. Published by the U.S. Department of Health and Human Services.

Hofmann, Regan. "The Same Old Me." *POZ,* November 2005, p.3.

Joint United Nations Programme on HIV/AIDS. "Urgent Response to the HIV/AIDS Epidemics in the Commonwealth of Independent States." Moscow, Russia. March 31–April 1 2005. Retrieved April 2006 (http://www.unodc.org/pdf/event_2005-03-31_young_people.pdf).

Kirby, D. "School-Based Interventions to Prevent Unprotected Sex and HIV Among Adolescents." *Handbook of HIV Prevention.* J. Peterson and R. Diclemente, eds. New York, NY: Plenum Publishers, 2000.

Lee, Alan. "Update on Vitamins & Minerals: What and How Much to Take." *HIV Positive,* June/July 2006, pp.28–31.

Lee, Susan. "Aids: Young People Dying of Embarrassment—HIV Report." Common Dreams News Center. Retrieved January 2006 (http://www.commondreams.org).

The National Campaign to Prevent Teen Pregnancy. "General Facts and Stats." Teenpregnancy.org. Retrieved August 2006 (http://www.teenpregnancy.org/resources/data/genlfact.asp).

New York State Department of Health. "Staying on Schedule: Taking Your HIV Medicines." February 2002.

UNAIDS/WHO AIDS Epidemic Update: December 2005. Retrieved July 2006 (http://www.unaids.org/epi/2005/doc/EPIupdate2005_html_en/epi05_03_en.htm).

United Nations General Assembly Special Session on HIV/AIDS. "Declaration of Commitment on HIV/AIDS: Global Targets for Young People, Dedicating Regional and World-Wide Efforts to Preventing HIV Transmission Among Young People." New York, NY. June 2001. Retrieved August 2006 (http://www.unaids.org/en/Goals/UNGASS/default.asp).

U.S. Department of Agriculture. "Inside the Pyramid." Mypyramid.gov. Retrieved August 2006 (http://www.mypyramid.gov/pyramid/index.html).

"Using Condoms, Condom Types & Condom Sizes." Avert.com. Retrieved August 2006 (http://www.avert.org/usecond.htm).

"What Is AIDS?" Centers for Disease Control and Prevention. Retrieved June 2006 (http://www.cdc.gov/hiv/resources/qa/qa2.htm).

White, Katherine. *Everything You Need to Know About AIDS and HIV.* New York, NY: The Rosen Publishing Group, 2001.

World Health Organization. "Global AIDS Statistics." *Global AIDS Focus AIDS Care,* Vol.8, No.2, pp.246–248. Retrieved August 2006 (http://taylorandfrancis.metapress.com/media/pf9gtmtwxrd97tmxcd4p/contributions/v/6/3/3/v633f8tc0a514087.pdf).

"Young People and AIDS." The Body: The Complete HIV/AIDS Resource at TheBody.com. Retrieved August 2006 (http://www.thebody.com/whatis/children.html).

"Zimbabwe Female Life Expectancy Falls to 34—Shortest in the World." *Sunday Telegraph,* reprinted in *Times-Colonist.* Victoria, BC, Canada. April 9, 2006, p.A10.

ABOUT THE AUTHOR

Paula Johanson has worked for twenty years as a writer and teacher, and she has written and edited curriculum educational materials for the Alberta Distance Learning Centre in Canada. This is her fourth book for Rosen Publishing. She writes and edits nonfiction books, magazine articles and columns, and book reviews. She has been nominated twice for the national Prix Aurora Award for Canadian Science Fiction. She had a blood transfusion in early 1985, before AIDS/HIV screening, but took an HIV test as soon as it was available. Ms. Johanson lives on an island in British Columbia and a farm in Alberta, Canada.

Photo Credits: Cover, © www.istockphoto.com.

Designer: Nelson Sà; Editor: Wayne Anderson

Back Cover Material

TITLES IN THIS SERIES

AVIAN FLU

BODY PIERCING AND TATTOOING
THE HIDDEN DANGERS OF BODY ART

HIV AND AIDS

OBESITY

STRESS

SUICIDE

T

U

V

W

Books For ALL Kinds of Readers

At ReadHowYouWant we understand that one size does not fit all types of readers. Our innovative, patent pending technology allows us to design new formats to make reading easier and more enjoyable for you. This helps improve your speed of reading and your comprehension. Our EasyRead printed books have been optimized to improve word recognition, ease eye tracking by adjusting word and line spacing as well as minimizing hyphenation. Our EasyRead SuperLarge editions have been developed to make reading easier and more accessible for vision-impaired readers. We offer Braille and DAISY formats of our books and all popular E-Book formats.

We are continually introducing new formats based upon research and reader preferences. Visit our web-site to see all of our formats and learn how you can Personalize our books for yourself or as gifts. Sign up to Become A RHYW Registered Reader.

www.readhowyouwant.com

Made in the USA
Monee, IL
05 November 2026

67811067R10077